HEALTHY LIVING

POST - LIVER TRANSPLANT DIET GUIDE &

COOKBOOK

Handy Liver Nutritional Guide.

By
CYNTHIA LEONARD

All rights reserved.

No part of this publication may be reproduced, distributed or transmitted in any form or by any means, including photocopying, recording or other electronic or mechanical methods, without prior written permission of the publisher, except in the case of brief quotations embodied in critical reviews and certain other non-commercial uses permitted by copyright law.

Copyright © [CYNTHIA LEONARD] 2023

TABLE OF CONTENTS

INTRO: HOW IMPORTANT DIET IS AFTER LIVER TRANSPLANTATION — 6

FINDING YOUR WAY THROUGH DIETARY CHANGES FOR A HEALTHY RECOVERY — 10

CHAPTER 1: — 15

THE BASICS OF A POST LIVER TRANSPLANT DIET — 15

NUTRITIONAL GOALS AND CONSIDERATIONS POST LIVER TRANSPLANT — 21

    Nutritional Objectives — 22

    Dietary Considerations — 24

MACRONUTRIENT BALANCE FOR OPTIMAL HEALING — 27

THE ROLE OF MICRONUTRIENTS IN IMMUNE SUPPORT — 30

CHAPTER 2: — 34

Transitioning to Solid Foods — 34

GRADUAL INTRODUCTION TO SOLID FOODS — 34

RECOMMENDED FOODS FOR INITIAL STAGES — 42

MONITORING DIGESTIVE TOLERANCE — 46

Gastrointestinal Changes Following Transplantation: 47

Monitoring indices: 47

Management and Intervention: 49

The significance of monitoring: 50

CHAPTER 3: 52

HYDRATION AND FLUID BALANCE 52

A Complete Guide on Hydration and Fluid Balance Following Liver Transplant 52

Guidelines for Hydration After Liver Transplant: 54

Dehydration and overhydration symptoms include: 56

FLUID INTAKE GUIDELINES AND MANAGING FLUID RETENTION 57

When to Seek Medical Attention and Warning Signs: 61

CHAPTER 4: 65

MANAGING MEDICATIONS AND NUTRITION 65

Interactions Between Immunosuppressants and Diet 65

TIMING MEALS WITH MEDICATION SCHEDULE 69

CHAPTER 5: 72

FOODS TO LIMIT OR AVOID	**72**
FOODS TO EMBRACE IN YOUR DIET	**75**
CHAPTER 6:	**81**
DEALING WITH DIGESTIVE ISSUES	**81**
Probiotics and Gut Health Support:	81
RECIPES:	**86**
QUICK AND EASY RECIPES FOR BUSY DAYS	**86**
BREAKFAST AND BRUNCH RECIPES	**91**
LUNCH AND DINNER RECIPES	**100**
Lunch Meals:	100
Dinner Meals:	113
SNACKS, SMOOTHIES AND DESSERTS	**126**
Snacks Meals:	126
Smoothie Meals:	131
Dessert Meals:	135
Bonus Recipes:	140

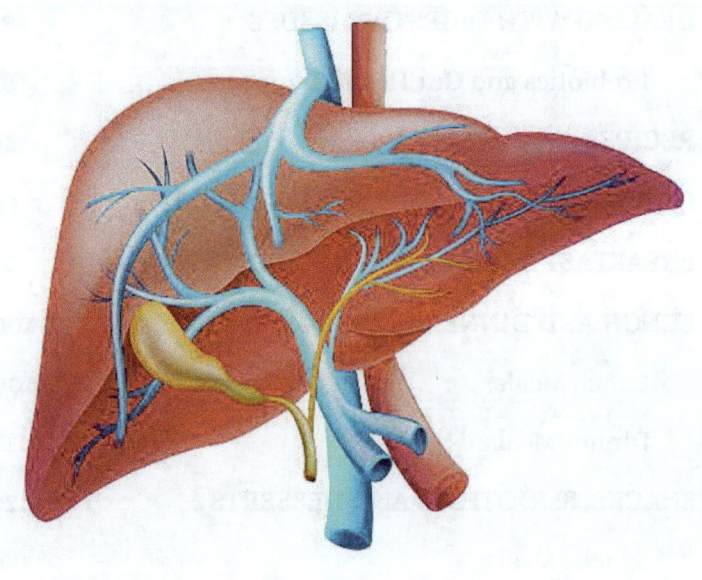

INTRO: HOW IMPORTANT DIET IS AFTER LIVER TRANSPLANTATION

Maintaining a nutritious diet after a liver transplant is essential for the procedure's success and the patient's general wellbeing. A healthy, balanced diet may benefit in a number of ways.

Supporting Healing and Recovery: Because a liver transplant is a significant medical surgery, the body needs the right nutrients to heal and recover. A healthy, protein- and vitamin-rich diet may help with tissue healing and general recuperation.

Preventing Infections and Complications: Following a liver transplant, immunosuppressive drugs are often administered to stop the body from rejecting the new organ. These drugs may lower immunological function, increasing the risk of infection for the patient. An immune system boost and decreased risk of infections may be achieved with a balanced diet that includes foods high in vitamins and antioxidants.

Taking Care of Your Medicines: Certain foods and nutrients may interfere with immunosuppressive treatments and other post-transplant medications. Making sure that the food does not affect the drugs and their absorption may be accomplished by carefully collaborating with a qualified dietitian.

Keeping Weight Gain to a Minimum: Some people may gain weight following a liver transplant as a result of things like medication side effects and metabolic changes. A diet that emphasises portion management, nutritional balance, and regular exercise may help avoid uncontrollable weight gain.

Preventing Metabolic Disorders: Metabolic disorders including diabetes and high cholesterol may affect liver transplant patients. A diet reduced in added sugars, processed carbs, and saturated and trans fats may help reduce these risks.

Maintaining Nutrient Levels: Due to the changed function of the donated liver, liver transplant patients may have difficulties absorbing certain nutrients. Deficiencies may be avoided by monitoring nutritional levels and changing the diet appropriately.

Liver Health: By lowering the risk of fatty liver disease and other disorders that might affect liver function, a balanced diet can promote the general health of the transplanted liver.

Hydration: Maintaining appropriate hydration is important for general health and may help the liver perform its duties. Digestion, detoxification, and the removal of waste from the body are all made easier by water.

Bone Health: Immunosuppressive drugs may have an impact on bone health, which can result in diseases like osteoporosis. Calcium and vitamin D-rich foods may support bone density maintenance.

Psychological Health: A liver transplant might result in major lifestyle adjustments and mental difficulties. A balanced diet may have a good effect on mood and general psychological health.

Working closely with a certified dietician with expertise in transplant nutrition is crucial for liver transplant patients. Based on the patient's medical history, current medicines, dietary preferences and any particular difficulties they may be experiencing, these experts may provide tailored advice. Following medical instructions, maintaining a healthy lifestyle, and eating the right foods may all help with liver transplant recovery and quality of life.

FINDING YOUR WAY THROUGH DIETARY CHANGES FOR A HEALTHY RECOVERY

Making deliberate decisions to support your body's healing process and general wellbeing is important while navigating dietary adjustments for a good recovery. Here are some tips to take into account whether you're recuperating from a disease or surgery or just trying to enhance your health:

1. Speak with a medical expert:

It's essential to speak with a healthcare expert, such as a doctor, registered dietitian, or nutritionist, before making any substantial dietary adjustments. They may provide you individualised guidance based on your unique health situation, dietary requirements, and objectives.

2. Put an emphasis on nutrient-dense foods:

Give nutrient-rich foods a higher priority since they include vital vitamins, minerals, and antioxidants. Fruits, vegetables, whole grains, lean proteins (such as chicken, fish, tofu, and lentils), nuts, seeds, and healthy fats (such as avocado and olive oil) are some examples of these.

3. Getting Enough Protein:

Protein is necessary for tissue regeneration and repair. Include sources of high-quality protein in your diet, such as quinoa, tofu, lean poultry, fish, eggs, dairy products, and lean meats, poultry, and legumes.

4. Water intake

All body processes, including healing, are supported by proper hydration. Consider hydrating meals such as soups, broths and fruits with a high water content as well as drinking water often throughout the day.

Omega-3 Fatty Acids (5):

Omega-3 fatty acids are anti-inflammatory and may help the body recover itself. Include sources in your diet such as flaxseeds, chia seeds, walnuts, and fatty fish *(salmon, mackerel and sardines)*.

6. Foods High in Fibre:

Both digestion and blood sugar levels are supported by fibre. To achieve a sufficient intake of dietary fibre, include whole grains, fruits, vegetables, legumes and seeds in your diet.

7. Limit processed food intake:

Reduce your intake of highly processed meals, sweet snacks, and foods with plenty of bad fats. These may cause inflammation and impede the healing process.

8. Take into account micronutrients:

For healing and rehabilitation, a few vitamins and minerals are very crucial. The immune system is supported by zinc, collagen creation is aided by vitamin C, and bone health is influenced by vitamin D. Include a range of these nutrients-rich foods in your diet.

9. Tiny, Regular Meals:

Consider eating smaller, more frequent meals if your appetite is low while you're recovering to make sure you're receiving all the nutrients you need without taxing your digestive system.

10. Organise special dietary requirements:

Work with a healthcare expert to customise your diet if you have any unique dietary needs or diseases *(such as allergies or diabetes)*.

11. Observe Portion Sizes:

Pay close attention to portion proportions to avoid eating too much or too little. Depending on your exercise level, metabolism, and state of health, you may have different calorie demands.

12. Gradual Alterations:

When switching to a new eating plan, it's extremely important to implement nutritional adjustments gradually. This strategy may assist your body in adjusting and lower the likelihood of pain.

CHAPTER 1:

THE BASICS OF A POST LIVER TRANSPLANT DIET

A significant medical operation known as a liver transplant includes replacing a sick or damaged liver with a healthy liver from a donor. Following a post-transplant diet is essential to promote healing, guarantee the success of the transplant, and preserve general health after a liver transplant. The fundamentals of a post-liver transplant diet are as follows:

Progressive Graduation:

Your diet will gradually transition from clear liquids to solid meals after the procedure. Your body can adapt and repair at its own speed thanks to this process.

2. Well-balanced Diet:

A balanced diet is crucial for general health and recovery. A balance of carbs, proteins, good fats, vitamins, and minerals should be included in your diet.

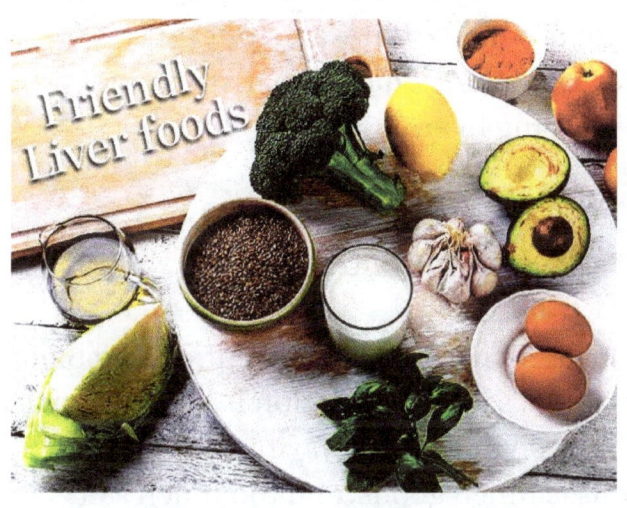

3. Protein Consumption

Protein is crucial for immune system health, muscular mass preservation and repair. Include lean protein sources in your diet, such as chicken, turkey, fish, beans, lentils, tofu and dairy products.

4. Fluid Consumption:

Maintaining organ function and avoiding problems require maintaining hydration. Drink adequate fluids, but watch out for overhydration, which might stress the developing liver.

5. Salt (Sodium) Control:

In order to control fluid retention and blood pressure, salt consumption has to be restricted. When cooking, stay away from processed foods, canned goods, and too much salt.

6. Consuming Fat:

Include wholesome fats from foods like olive oil, nuts, seeds, and avocados. Steer clear of the saturated and trans fats that may be found in fatty meats, pastries, and fried meals.

7. Foods High in Fibre:

Fibre helps avoid constipation and supports digestive health. To boost your intake of fibre, eat whole grains, fruits, vegetables, and legumes.

8. Supplementing with vitamins and minerals:

Your medical staff may advise vitamin and mineral supplements, such as calcium, vitamin D, vitamin B12, and iron, due to possible nutritional shortages.

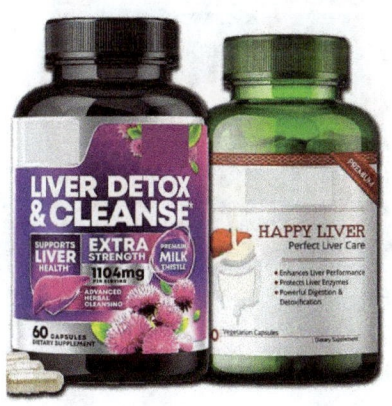

9. Avoid too much sugar and sweets:

Reduce your consumption of sweetened meals and drinks. Consuming too much sugar may lead to weight gain and other health problems.

10. Avoiding alcohol:

After a liver transplant, alcohol use is normally discouraged since it might strain the new liver more and affect how well medications work.

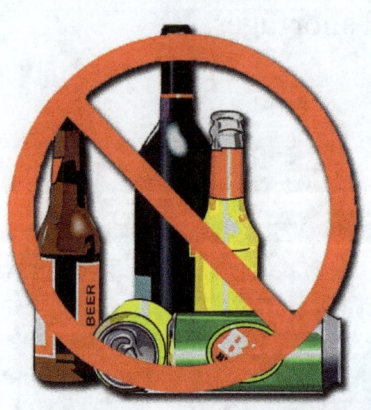

11. Drug Interactions:

Be mindful of possible interactions between specific meals and the prescription drugs you take after a transplant. To learn about any limits or safety measures, speak with your medical team or a qualified nutritionist.

12. Individualised Strategy:

Keep in mind that each person's dietary requirements might change depending on things like age, weight, medical history, and medicines. To create a custom post-transplant nutrition plan, work closely with your medical team and a licensed dietitian.

13. Consistent Monitoring:

Your transplant team will be able to track your progress and change your diet and medication as needed via routine follow-up sessions.

A nutritious post-liver transplant diet strives to enhance your quality of life, help the recovery process and avert problems.

NUTRITIONAL GOALS AND CONSIDERATIONS POST LIVER TRANSPLANT

An unhealthy or dysfunctional liver is replaced with a healthy liver from a dead or living donor during a complicated surgical process known as a liver transplant. People with end-stage liver disease, acute liver failure, or specific malignancies connected to the liver often need this life-saving procedure. The post-transplant phase requires meticulous attention to several areas of the patient's health, including **diet**, even though the surgical success is vital.

A liver transplant is followed by a time period during which there are considerable physiological and metabolic changes. The patient's dietary requirements, nutrient absorption and general wellbeing may all be negatively impacted by these changes. To guarantee the patient's recovery, immunological function, wound healing and

Problems prevention, it is crucial to set suitable dietary objectives and considerations.

Nutritional Objectives

Promote Healing and Recovery: The body goes through a significant healing and tissue regeneration process after surgery. To support these processes and guarantee a speedy recovery, adequate diet is vital and should include protein, vitamins, and other essential nutrients.

Maintain Lean Body Mass: To avoid rejection of the new liver after transplant, the immune system's performance is crucial. Protein is essential for boosting immune system health and avoiding muscle atrophy. In order to retain lean body mass, it is essential to maintain a sufficient protein consumption.

Reduce the Risk of Infection:
Immunosuppressive drugs are recommended after organ transplantation to avoid organ rejection. Nevertheless, they also impair immunity, leaving patients more prone to infections. Infection risks may be reduced with a proper diet, which is rich in vitamins and minerals that promote immunological function.

Manage Medication Interactions: Some foods may interfere with the absorption or efficacy of immunosuppressive drugs. To promote the best possible performance of the drugs, nutritional planning should take these interactions into account.

Preventing metabolic complications: This is important because patients who get organ transplants may have changes in their metabolism, including insulin resistance, hyperlipidemia, and bone loss. To avoid these issues, a balanced diet that controls lipid profiles, blood sugar levels, and bone health is crucial.

Dietary Considerations

Calculating the proper calorie intake is essential for avoiding under- or overeating. Age, gender, amount of physical activity and general health state may all affect calorie needs.

Consuming protein is essential for immunological health, muscle maintenance, and wound healing. Consuming enough protein is important, but not too much protein might stress the liver.

Micronutrient Supplementation:
Post-transplant, deficiencies in some vitamins and minerals, including vitamin D, calcium, and magnesium, may arise from drugs, insufficient sun exposure, or abnormal absorption. Monitoring and supplementation on a regular basis may assist keep levels at their ideal.

Hydration: Because immunosuppressive drugs are often used by transplant patients, adequate hydration improves kidney function and helps avoid problems like kidney stones.

Diet that is well-balanced: A diet high in fruits, vegetables, whole grains, and lean meats supplies necessary nutrients while promoting gut health, which is strongly related to immune system performance as a whole.

Restricting your salt consumption might help you avoid fluid retention and high blood pressure. Intake of salt should be restricted since people who have had liver transplants are susceptible to these problems.

Consuming fat with caution: Dyslipidemia might be a risk for transplant patients. It is advised to choose healthy fats, such as those in nuts, seeds and fatty fish.

Avoid drinking alcohol since it may strain the liver and affect how medications are metabolised. Alcohol abstinence is required of all post-transplant patients.

Regular Monitoring: During the post-transplant journey, nutritional demands may change. To accommodate shifting demands, nutritional evaluations and modifications must be made often.

Personalization: Each transplant patient is different, and depending on their medical history and the particulars of their transplant, they may have different dietary requirements. For best results, trained dietitians should collaborate on the creation of individualised nutrition regimens.

The patient's general health and speedy recovery depend greatly on the dietary objectives and considerations they make following a liver transplant. A balanced diet that is tailored to the requirements of the individual may promote healing, support the immune system and ward against difficulties.

MACRONUTRIENT BALANCE FOR OPTIMAL HEALING

The best healing and recovery after a liver transplant need close attention to many different elements of your health, including diet. Macronutrient balancing is a vital part of post-transplant treatment since it has an immediate influence on your body's capacity to recover, regenerate tissues and promote general health. Following a liver transplant, balance your macronutrient intake for the best healing potential are -

Consumption of protein is crucial for immune system health, tissue healing and sustaining muscular mass. Protein is even more important after a liver transplant because it helps the body repair surgical wounds and maintain liver tissue regrowth. Include lean protein sources in your diet, such as chicken, fish, eggs, dairy, lentils and tofu. For individualised recommendations, speak with your medical team and aim for 1.2 to 1.5 grams of protein per kilogramme of body weight each day.

Meanwhile carbohydrates provide your body energy to power its recuperative mechanisms and stop muscular deterioration. Put an emphasis on foods with complex carbs, such as whole grains, fruits, vegetables and legumes. These energy sources give prolonged energy for recovery and slowly release energy, both of which contribute to stable blood sugar levels.

Healthy fats are essential for cellular function, inflammation reduction, and the absorption of fat-soluble vitamins. Avocados, almonds, seeds, olive oil, and fatty fish *(such salmon and mackerel)* are good sources of unsaturated fats. The omega-3 fatty acids in fish oil are anti-inflammatory and may aid in healing.

Your body's transportation of nutrients, circulation and digestion are all supported by water. Drink plenty of water throughout the day, and think about including foods that are high in water in your meals.

Getting enough vitamins and minerals is important for a number of biological processes, including as immune support and wound healing. To guarantee you're receiving a variety of nutrients, put an emphasis on a varied selection of colourful fruits and vegetables. You could also think about taking vitamin and mineral supplements if your medical staff advises them to treat any deficiencies.

Take small, regular meals because liver transplant may cause your body's metabolic rate to change. Consider consuming fewer, smaller meals more often throughout the day rather than three big ones. In addition to supporting digestion and ensuring a consistent supply of nutrients for healing, this strategy may help keep blood sugar levels stable.

Consult with your doctor, particularly after a major medical surgery like a liver transplant, each person has specific dietary demands. Based on your medical history, present condition and any medicines you are currently taking, your healthcare team, which includes dietitians and physicians, will provide personalised advice. Also discuss your progress with your medical team. They may monitor your nutritional status, correct any issues, and modify your diet and macronutrient intake as needed according to how your body is reacting to the transplant.

THE ROLE OF MICRONUTRIENTS IN IMMUNE SUPPORT

Micronutrients are essential for sustaining general health and boosting the immune system's operation. The body needs these crucial vitamins and minerals in minute levels for a variety of physiological activities, including immunological response. Here is a summary of several important micronutrients and how they boost the immune system:

Vitamin C: This anti-oxidant is well-known for strengthening the immune system. It promotes the development and operation of different immune cells, including white blood cells.

Additionally, vitamin C encourages the synthesis of antibodies and assists in preventing oxidative stress from damaging immune cells.

Vitamin D: Also known as the "sunshine vitamin," vitamin D is essential for the immune system to operate properly. It stimulates the growth and activation of immune cells and aids in controlling the immunological response. Infection susceptibility has been linked to vitamin D deficiency in studies.

Vitamin A is necessary for preserving the health of the skin and mucous membranes, which serve as defences against microorganisms. Additionally, it aids in the regulation of the immune response and the growth of immune cells.

Vitamin E: This antioxidant vitamin maintains the health and function of immune cells by assisting in the prevention of oxidative damage. Additionally, it increases antibody synthesis and fortifies the body's defence systems.

Zinc: Zinc has a role in a number of immunological functions, such as the growth and operation of immune cells. It is essential for controlling inflammation and a lack of it may make the immune system less effective. Additionally, zinc promotes wound healing and preserves the health of the skin and mucous membranes.

Selenium: This mineral is necessary for the creation of selenoproteins, which function as immunological regulators and have antioxidant qualities. Lack of selenium might weaken the immune system and make you more susceptible to diseases.

Iron: Iron is important for immune system health and for the creation of haemoglobin, which carries oxygen to cells. Anaemia brought on by iron shortage may impair the immune system's capacity to react.

Copper: Copper contributes to immune cell growth and function as well as the development of connective tissues that promote immunological function. Additionally, it possesses antioxidant qualities that aid in the defence of immunological cells against harm.

While these micronutrients are necessary for supporting the immune system, it's vital to remember that more is not always better. The goal is to keep up a diversified, balanced diet that contains plenty of foods high in nutrients. Getting these nutrients only from supplements may not be as advantageous as getting them from entire meals. Individual dietary requirements might differ depending on characteristics including age, sex, health state and degree of exercise.

CHAPTER 2:

Transitioning to Solid Foods

GRADUAL INTRODUCTION TO SOLID FOODS

Here is a broad strategy you may take into account:

Consult Your Medical Team: Always speak with your transplant surgeon, hepatologist or a registered dietitian with experience in post-transplant nutrition before making any dietary changes. They will be the most knowledgeable about your medical background and present state of health.

Timing: After a liver transplant, there is no set time for introducing solid meals. When you've made major strides in your recovery, your liver function is stable and your medical team gives you the all-clear, you may often begin introducing solid meals.

Start out slowly: Start with meals that are simple to digest and minimal risk. Examples include moderate grains like rice and oats, well-cooked veggies like carrots and peas, and well-cooked fruits like apples and pears. Digestional pain is less likely to be brought on by these meals.

Avoid High-Risk Foods: To start, stay away from foods that are prone to infection or are known to be difficult to digest. This may include unpasteurized dairy products, uncooked eggs, undercooked meat, and raw or undercooked shellfish.

Water intake: Maintaining enough water intake is essential for general health and post-transplant recovery. Drink plenty of water throughout the day to be well hydrated, which will help with digestion and general wellbeing.

Portion control: Start with modest quantities when reintroducing solid meals to give your body time to become used to processing and digesting them once again. Your digestive system won't have to work as hard, thanks to this.

Allergies and Tolerance: Keep an eye out for food intolerances or allergies by paying attention to how your body responds to various meals. Even after a transplant, allergic reactions or dietary intolerances might still happen. Inform your medical staff if you experience any negative side effects.

A balanced diet that includes a range of nutrient-rich foods should be gradually attained. Your healing and general health may be supported by consuming fruits, vegetables, lean meats, whole grains and healthy fats.

Avoid Overloading Your Liver: Even if your new liver is operating properly, it's important to avoid providing it with too many nutrients, particularly too much salt and sugar. Modesty is important.

Follow-up visits should be made on a regular basis to check on your general health and liver function. Depending on how you're doing, your medical team may change the diet suggestions they've made.

Keep in mind that these recommendations are broad in nature and may not be applicable to all situations.

A Spelled out description of the progressive introduction of solid meals following a liver transplant in detail:

First Step: Medical Clearance

Your medical team will evaluate your general health, liver function, and post-transplant recovery status before you start introducing solid meals. They will give you the go-ahead to begin the process of switching to solid meals once they determine it is suitable.

Consult a registered Dietitian:

A certified dietician with expertise in post-transplant nutrition should be consulted. They will work with you to develop a strategy that is unique to your requirements, medical background, and nutritional choices.

Start using foods that are Simple to Digest:

Start with items that are simple on the stomach. These might consist of soft, well prepared vegetables *(such as carrots and peas)*, properly prepared fruits (such as ap*ples and pears)*, and light grains *(such as rice and oats)*. Digestional pain is less likely to be brought on by these meals.

Introduce One New food at a time:

One novel dish at a time should be introduced. This enables you to keep track of how your body reacts to various foods and aids in the detection of any possible allergies or intolerances.

Monitor for Reactions:

Keep a watchful eye on your body's response after introducing a new cuisine. Keep an eye out for any indications of stomach pain, intolerances or allergies. If you have any negative consequences, stop eating that meal and seek medical advice.

Gradually Expand the Variety of Food:

Expand your diet variety gradually as your body gets used to eating solid foods again. Your diet should include a variety of fruits, vegetables, lean meats, entire grains and healthy fats. Still, keep away from risky items like raw shellfish and underdone meats.

Controlling portions:

To avoid your digestive system from being overloaded, start with tiny meals. In time, as your body becomes used to digesting solid meals, you may increase portion sizes.

Continue to hydrate:

Make sure you're getting enough water each day. Drinking enough water stimulates digestion, prevents constipation and enhances general health.

Consistent Medical Checkups:

Keep going to your regular doctor's checkups to keep an eye on your general health and liver function. Based on your success and any changes in your medical condition, your medical team may revise the diet suggestions they have made for you.

Listen to your body:

Pay attention to how your body responds to various meals. Inform your medical staff if you feel any pain, bloating, or other unexpected symptoms.

Gradual Development:

You may gradually make the switch to a more diverse and balanced diet as your body adjusts to solid meals and your recovery progresses. But always put your health first and heed the advice of your medical staff.

RECOMMENDED FOODS FOR INITIAL STAGES

Following a liver transplant, it's crucial to concentrate on eating meals that are simple to digest, soft on the liver, and rich in nutrients that the body needs to mend and recover. Here are some possible suggestions:

Start with fruits that are simple to digest, such as mashed bananas, ripe pears and applesauce. These may provide natural sugars, fibre and vitamins.

Steamed or boiled veggies like carrots, sweet potatoes and zucchini may be easy on the stomach. Start by avoiding veggies with a lot of fibre. Consider well cooked cereals like muesli and rice. They provide some fibre and energy without unduly taxing the digestive system.

Introduce lean protein sources gradually, such as cooked chicken, turkey or mild fish. These are crucial for muscle preservation and recovery.

Mild cheeses or plain yoghurt might provide some protein as well as healthy bacteria for the intestines. Make sure to choose low-fat choices if your medical staff suggests them.

Soups and broths made from lean meats and properly prepared vegetables may provide hydration and nutrients.

You may also add a little bit of healthy fat to your meals, such as avocado or olive oil. Both energy and nutrition absorption may benefit from them. It's crucial to maintain hydration for healing. As tolerated, sip on water, herbal teas and diluted fruit juices.

Avoid Strong Spices and Seasonings as It's advisable to stay away from highly seasoned meals in the beginning since they could be difficult for your body to tolerate.

Instead of eating three or four substantial meals during the day, consider eating small, frequent meals. This may help keep the digestive system from being overworked.

Keep track of how your body reacts to various meals. Consider altering your diet and seeking the advice of your healthcare team if you experience any pain, bloating or other negative responses.

It's crucial to make sure you're receiving enough vitamins and minerals while you're healing. To remedy any nutritional shortages, your healthcare staff may suggest a multivitamin or certain supplements.

You may gradually increase your intake of foods high in fibre, such as cooked vegetables, whole grains and fruits, while your digestive system adapts. Increase your fibre intake gradually to avoid any discomfort.

Protein is essential for muscle repair and maintenance. Several different lean protein foods, such as chicken, fish, tofu, lentils and dairy products *(if permitted)*, should be included into your diet.

Limiting processed meals may help your liver, which may have a tougher time processing overly processed and fried foods. Whenever possible, choose whole, minimally processed foods and keep an eye on your salt intake since too much sodium might cause fluid retention. Consider consuming less salt and opting for low-sodium or salt-free choices.

Be careful while resuming foods if you have any known food allergies or intolerances. Your medical staff may advise you on when and how to safely reintroduce them.

Slowly increase the diversity of foods in your diet over time. Pay attention to how your body reacts and adjust as necessary.

Avoid Alcohol since it may mix with drugs and put extra pressure on the liver. Your medical team will probably plan routine examinations and testing to keep track of your general health and liver function. Use these meetings to address any dietary questions you may have and to seek advice on your diet strategy.

Flexibility and patience are required since recovery is a slow process and you may need to adjust your diet as you go. Be kind to your body and yourself and be willing to change your diet as necessary.

MONITORING DIGESTIVE TOLERANCE

Monitoring digestive tolerance after a liver transplant, while consuming solid meals is an essential part of postoperative treatment. Patients' digestive systems may undergo substantial alterations after surgery as a result of things like changed bile flow, possible complications and the effects of immunosuppressive drugs. In order to maintain optimal nutritional absorption, avoid problems and aid the patient's overall recovery, regular monitoring of digestive tolerance is crucial.

Gastrointestinal Changes Following Transplantation:

Digestive tolerance may alter as a result of numerous gastrointestinal changes brought on by liver transplantation. Bile is produced by the liver and helps in the digestion and absorption of fat. After a transplant, altered bile flow might cause problems with fat digestion, which can cause malabsorption and diarrhoea. The gastrointestinal system's functionality may also be impacted by the surgical process itself, the use of immunosuppressant and possible side effects such as graft rejection.

Monitoring indices:

Dietary Progression: From clear liquids to solid meals, the patient's diet is steadily progressing. This evaluates the patient's tolerance for various meal textures and compositions and enables the gastrointestinal system to adjust to the changes.

Nutrient Intake: It's essential to keep track of the patient's calorie and nutrient intake to avoid malnutrition. For wound healing, immune system health, and general recovery, high-quality proteins, vitamins and minerals are crucial.

Faeces characteristics: Examining the regularity, consistency, and colour of the faeces reveals information about digestive process. The presence of loose stools, oily stools, or changes in stool colour may be signs of problems with fat absorption.

Gastrointestinal symptoms, including nausea, vomiting, bloating, gas and stomach pain, are kept an eye on in patients. These signs might point to digestive issues or consequences including transplant rejection.

Weight fluctuations: Regular weight checks assist spot sudden weight gain or decrease, pointing to possible malabsorption or fluid retention problems.

Management and Intervention:

Dietary Modification: The dietician may change the patient's nutritional intake in accordance with the patient's digestive tolerance. To enable proper digestion and absorption, this may include changing the ratio of fats, proteins and carbs in the diet.

Digestive enzyme supplements may be administered to help with nutrition absorption and fat digestion. Lipase supplements may aid in the breakdown of lipids, hence easing the symptoms of malabsorption.

Fluid and electrolyte balance: Vomiting and diarrhoea may cause an imbalance in these two elements. It is vital to keep an eye on these levels and provide any required treatments, such restoration of lost electrolytes and fluids.

Immunosuppressive medicine is used to avoid organ rejection, however it has the potential to cause gastrointestinal adverse effects. To preserve general health, it's crucial to closely monitor these side effects and, if required, make prescription modifications.

The significance of monitoring:

Malnutrition must be avoided since it may impair a patient's ability to recover and their immune system. This can be done by ensuring that nutrients are properly digested and absorbed.

Complications may be identified early thanks to gastrointestinal symptoms, which can also signal graft rejection or other problems. An early intervention may stop things from becoming worse.

Enhancing Quality of Life: During the recovery period, the patient's overall comfort and quality of life are improved by effective control of digestive tolerance.

Personalised Care: The way that solid meals affect each patient's digestive system varies. Monitoring enables individually customised actions to meet each person's requirements.

Surgeons, nutritionists, nurses and other healthcare professionals must work closely together to monitor digestive tolerance throughout the consumption of solid meals following a liver transplant. It seeks to guarantee the patient's capacity for efficient nutrition absorption and digestion, avoid problems and encourage successful post-transplant recovery. Medical practitioners are able to respond quickly with the proper steps to improve the patient's digestive health and general well-being by carefully monitoring metrics including dietary progression, nutrient intake, stool characteristics, gastrointestinal symptoms and weight changes.

CHAPTER 3:

HYDRATION AND FLUID BALANCE

A Complete Guide on Hydration and Fluid Balance Following Liver Transplant

A sophisticated surgical operation called a liver transplant includes swapping out a damaged or dysfunctional liver with a healthy donor liver. Maintaining correct hydration and fluid balance is essential for the patient's general recovery and well-being after such a big medical intervention. The liver's functioning may be impacted by the transplant since it is crucial for controlling the body's fluid balance. This tutorial will discuss the significance of fluid balance and hydration after liver transplantation as well as practical tips to guarantee a speedy recovery.

The Value of Fluid Balance and Hydration

The equilibrium of the body's fluid intake and outflow is known as fluid balance. By manufacturing proteins that control fluid flow between blood arteries and the tissues around them, the liver plays a crucial part in preserving this equilibrium. Due to modifications in liver function and drugs, the body of the patient may undergo changes in fluid dynamics after a liver transplant. Unbalances brought on by these alterations may hinder the patient's recuperation.

Post-liver transplant difficulties:

Edema: Modified protein synthesis in the liver may result in edema or the buildup of fluid in tissues. Swelling, pain, and possible consequences might result from this. Hydration is important in reducing excessive fluid retention.

Imbalance in electrolytes: The liver is in charge of processing electrolytes including sodium, potassium, and chloride. These electrolyte levels may become unbalanced after a transplant, which might impact muscle contractions, neuron signalling and heart function. Consuming enough liquids helps keep these vital electrolyte levels stable.

Immunosuppressant medicines are often required by patients to stop organ rejection. Some of these drugs may affect renal function and fluid balance. Monitoring your water levels carefully may help stop negative consequences.

Guidelines for Hydration After Liver Transplant:

Consult Your Medical Team: When it comes to your hydration consumption, heed the advice of your medical team. They will take into account your unique medical history, prescriptions and any particular requirements you may have.

Keep an eye on your urine production as you monitor your fluid intake. Dehydration may be indicated by a reduction in urine production. Urine that is clear to light yellow often suggests adequate hydration.

Intake of Fluids: Aim to consume enough fluids throughout the day. The ideal option is water, but you may also add herbal teas, clear broths and diluted fruit juices. Steer clear of beverages with a lot of sugar and caffeine.

Consume foods high in electrolytes, such as bananas *(potassium)*, spinach *(magnesium)* and avocados *(sodium)*, to maintain a healthy balance of electrolytes. These could support keeping the electrolyte equilibrium.

Reduce Your Sodium Intake: Too much sodium might cause fluid retention. Choose natural foods over processed and salty snacks.

Increase Gradually: If you have trouble with fluid retention, work with your medical team to gradually increase your fluid intake while keeping an eye on the results.

Avoid Overhydration: While enough hydration is important, avoid overhydration since this may stress your kidneys and throw off the balance of your electrolytes.

Dehydration and overhydration symptoms include:

Dehydration is characterised by dark yellow urine, dry mouth, thirst, dry skin, lightheadedness and a strong urine odour. If you encounter these symptoms, drink more water and speak with your doctor.

Overhydration may cause swelling in the limbs, rapid weight gain, breathlessness and weariness. Consult your medical provider right away if you have any of these symptoms.

Maintaining hydration and fluid balance is crucial for a quick recovery after a liver transplant due to the intricate interactions between liver function, medications, and fluid dynamics. Monitoring fluid intake and output and recognizing dehydration or overhydration symptoms can significantly improve overall well-being and transplant success. Healthcare specialists should be consulted for personalised assistance, as each individual's circumstances are unique.

FLUID INTAKE GUIDELINES AND MANAGING FLUID RETENTION

Guidelines for Fluid Intake:

Individualised Approach: Depending on a patient's age, weight, medical history, and the particular surgical operation, fluid intake recommendations may change from patient to patient. In order to meet the particular patient demands, an individualised strategy is necessary.

Hydration: Maintaining organ function, wound healing, and general health all depend on getting enough water into the body. To prevent both dehydration and overhydration, patients should strive to drink a balanced quantity of fluids.

Water: The main fluid source and the basis of fluid intake should be water. The best options are clear liquids like water, herbal teas and diluted fruit juices.

Electrolyte Balance: The maintenance of fluid balance depends heavily on electrolytes like sodium, potassium, and chloride. Fluid intake may be regulated by paying attention to electrolyte levels and following medical experts' recommendations.

Avoid Too Much Sugar and Caffeine: Too much sugar and caffeine may cause electrolyte imbalances and dehydration. Patients should avoid drinking too much caffeine and sugary drinks.

Monitoring urine output may provide information about your level of hydration. Dehydration may be indicated by urine that is dark or scarce, whereas overhydration may be indicated by urine that is too light.

Following a liver transplant, managing fluid retention:

After a liver transplant, fluid retention, also known as edema, may happen for a number of reasons. Controlling fluid retention is crucial for avoiding concerns including infection, sluggish wound healing and respiratory problems.

Medication Management: Immunosuppressive drugs that transplant recipients take may cause fluid retention. To lessen this impact, doctors may change the dose of the medicine.

Modifications to the diet: A low-sodium *(low-salt)* diet may aid in lowering fluid retention. Patients should avoid processed meals, canned soups, and salty snacks as high-sodium foods might cause water retention.

Elevate Legs: Lower extremity edema may be lessened by elevating the legs when relaxing or sleeping. This facilitates the body's removal of extra fluid from the legs.

Compression Clothing: By enhancing blood circulation, compression stockings or clothing may help avoid the accumulation of fluid in the legs.

Exercise regularly: As recommended by medical specialists, mild exercise may assist to increase blood circulation and decrease fluid retention.

Regular Follow-Ups: It's important to schedule regular post-transplant follow-up meetings with medical professionals. They may keep an eye on fluid retention, change medicines and provide the patient specific advice depending on their situation.

Monitor Weight: Patients should periodically check their weight, ideally at the same time every day and should notify their medical staff of any sudden or major changes. Gaining weight quickly might be a sign of fluid retention.

Avoid Drinking Too Much Fluid: While proper hydration is important, drinking too much fluid might make fluid retention worse. It's crucial to adhere to the suggested fluid consumption recommendations.

Psychosocial Support: It's important to recognise that the time after a liver transplant may be emotionally and physically taxing. Patients may feel stressed, anxious or other feelings as a result of the procedure and the subsequent recuperation. These mental conditions may affect fluid retention. As a result, it is beneficial to include psychological assistance in the patient's treatment strategy. *This might include family involvement in the healing process, support groups and counselling*.

When to Seek Medical Attention and Warning Signs:

Patients should be aware of any possible warning symptoms that might point to a more severe problem when treating fluid retention.

The following symptoms should be taken seriously and need immediate medical attention:

Weight Gain That Is Sudden and Significant: Sudden and significant weight gain should be reported to medical specialists since it may indicate fluid retention.

Edema that is severe enough to cause discomfort, pain, or trouble moving about needs medical attention.

Breathing Problems: Breathing problems or increasing shortness of breath, particularly while laying down, may be signs of pleural effusion, a condition where fluid builds up around the lungs.

Chest discomfort: Severe cardiac or pulmonary conditions may be indicated by persistent chest discomfort, especially when it is accompanied by shortness of breath.

Reduced Urine production: Urine production that suddenly drops off may be a sign of renal problems and needs to be evaluated by a doctor.

Ongoing Partnership with Healthcare Professionals:

Fluid management and fluid retention avoidance are continual procedures that need cooperation from the patient, carers and medical staff. For the purpose of keeping track of the patient's development and making any required modifications to the treatment plan, regular follow-up consultations with doctors and transplant coordinators are essential.

Education and empowerment: It is crucial to educate patients and carers about the significance of fluid management and how it affects post-transplant recovery. Giving patients the information they need to make informed decisions about their food, hydration consumption and self-monitoring may improve results and speed up the healing process.

After a liver transplant, rehabilitation requires commitment, knowledge and a holistic approach that takes into account one's physical, emotional and medical needs. A crucial part of post-liver transplant therapy is fluid control. Individualised fluid intake recommendations and methods for controlling fluid retention are essential to a complete recovery and the avoidance of problems.

CHAPTER 4:

MANAGING MEDICATIONS AND NUTRITION

Interactions Between Immunosuppressants and Diet

Immunosuppressant interactions with diet must be taken into account since particular meals and dietary practices may affect the efficiency and security of these drugs. Immunosuppressants are often recommended to treat autoimmune illnesses, organ transplants, and certain inflammatory conditions in order to stop the immune system from attacking the body's own tissues. *Following are some basic suggestions to remember when it comes to immunosuppressants and diet*:

Citrus fruits, especially grapefruit and several others, may interact with a number of drugs, including immunosuppressants. They include substances that prevent liver enzymes from metabolising medications, which might result in greater blood levels of the medication. This might make adverse effects and toxicity more likely. If you're using immunosuppressant medication, it's typically advised to stay away from grapefruit and grapefruit juice.

Foods High in Vitamin K: Certain immunosuppressants, such as certain blood thinners *(anticoagulants)*, may interact with foods high in vitamin K, such as leafy greens *(such as spinach, kale and broccoli)*. These drugs may alter how your body uses vitamin K, which is important for blood clotting. While taking these drugs, it's crucial to maintain a regular diet of foods high in vitamin K and to collaborate with your doctor to track the efficacy of your prescription.

Calcium and dairy products: Some immunosuppressants, especially corticosteroids, might raise the chance of osteoporosis and bone loss. For healthy bones, calcium and vitamin D are necessary. However, certain immunosuppressants may have an impact on how well the body assimilates calcium. It's crucial to make sure you get enough calcium and vitamin D while taking these drugs from sources including fortified meals, leafy greens, and supplements, as advised by your doctor.

Some immunosuppressants may interact with alcohol, which might influence how the drug is metabolised and how well it works. Additionally, *alcohol may interact with some illnesses that call for immunosuppressants* and may have a deleterious impact on the immune system. It is advisable to talk with your healthcare practitioner about drinking.

High-Fiber Foods: Gastrointestinal problems may be a negative effect of several immunosuppressants. In certain situations, eating meals high in fibre may make these symptoms worse. Your doctor may advise changing your diet to include more meals that are simple to digest if you have digestive pain.

Consuming salt: Immunosuppressive medications can cause fluid retention and elevated blood pressure. Consuming less sodium *(salt)* may aid in the management of certain problems. Pay attention to processed foods and restaurant meals since they might contain a lot of salt.

Consuming protein: Protein is crucial for repairing and maintaining muscular mass. Certain immunosuppressants may have an impact on protein synthesis. To make sure you're receiving the right amount of protein depending on your medications and health condition, speak with a certified dietitian or other healthcare professional.

Be aware that every person reacts differently to drugs and food combinations. It's crucial to be upfront with your doctor and, if appropriate, a trained dietitian who can provide you individualised advice based on your unique medicines, medical history and dietary choices.

TIMING MEALS WITH MEDICATION SCHEDULE

It may be beneficial to time meals with medication regimens for a variety of reasons, particularly if you're taking medicines that must be taken under certain circumstances in order to be safe or effective. It's important to remember that I'm not a doctor and that you should always get advice on your medicine and meal time from your doctor or chemist. In light of that, the following are some basic suggestions to bear in mind:

Always abide by your healthcare provider's or the chemist's directions about how and when to take your drugs. While certain drugs should be taken on an empty stomach, others may need to be taken with food to reduce any possible adverse effects.

Food Interactions: Some medicines may interact with food, which may reduce their absorption or effectiveness. Some medicines should be taken on an empty stomach to ensure optimal absorption, while others need to be taken with food to soothe the stomach or improve absorption. Make careful to enquire with your doctor or chemist about any possible dietary interactions with the particular drugs you're taking.

Regular Routine: **Try to create a regular schedule for taking your prescriptions and eating meals. This may make it simpler for you to plan your meals and can also help you remember to take your medicine.**

Meal Timing for Blood Sugar Control: **If you have diabetes or are taking drugs that alter blood sugar levels, it is even more crucial to plan your meals around your medication schedule. For instance, timing your meals to coincide with your insulin dosage may be necessary if you use insulin to avoid blood sugar rises or falls.**

Medication Requirements: **Some medicines have particular guidelines about when to take them in relation to meals. For instance, it may be necessary to take antibiotics before or after** meals for a certain period of time. It's essential to adhere to these recommendations to make sure the drug performs as intended.

Adjustments for Special Diets: If you follow a special diet, such as a low-sodium or high-fibre diet, it's crucial to take your prescriptions into account. Some diets may impact how well a drug works or is absorbed.

Consult experts: Before beginning a new medicine, find out when it is best to take it in relation to meals from your doctor or chemist. Based on your prescriptions and current health, they may provide tailored advice.

Use alarms or medication reminder applications to help you remember to take your prescriptions on time and in conjunction with meals.

CHAPTER 5:

FOODS TO LIMIT OR AVOID

To promote the healing process, guarantee adequate liver function, and lower the risk of problems after a liver transplant, it's essential to eat a balanced, nutritious diet. Although each person's dietary requirements may differ, the following are some basic recommendations on what foods to restrict or stay away from after a liver transplant:

1. Foods high in Sodium: A diet heavy in sodium may cause fluid retention and high blood pressure, both of which can put stress on the liver. meals rich in salt, such as processed meals, canned soups, packaged snacks, and fast food, should be avoided.

2. Sweetened foods and drinks: A high sugar consumption might result in weight gain and insulin resistance. Steer clear of sweets, candies, and desserts, as well as sugar-sweetened beverages like soda, fruit juices, and energy drinks.

3. Heavy-Fat Foods: A diet heavy in fat may cause weight gain and fatty liver, which is bad for the health of the liver. Eat less fried meals, fatty meat, full-fat dairy and baked goods, which are rich in saturated and trans fats.

4. Alcohol: Drinking alcohol may tax the liver and obstruct the body's ability to break down medications. Following a liver transplant, it is advised to abstain from alcohol entirely.

5. Raw Seafood: Consuming raw seafood, such as oysters, clams, and sushi, might increase the chance of contracting an infection, especially in those whose immune systems have been compromised by immunosuppressive drugs used after organ transplantation.

6. Undercooked Meats and Eggs: To prevent foodborne infections, make sure that all meats and eggs are cooked thoroughly. For accurate inside temperatures, use a food thermometer.

7. Overly Spicy meals: Spicy meals might upset some people's stomachs or create other digestive problems after transplantation. Keep track of your body's reactions and modify your intake as necessary.

8. Grapefruit and grapefruit juice: Grapefruit and its juice may affect how several medicines, which are often used after a transplant, are metabolised, resulting in greater or lower blood levels of these drugs.

9. Foods rich in Vitamin K: If you use blood-thinning drugs like warfarin, you should exercise caution while eating foods rich in vitamin K, such as leafy greens *(spinach, kale, and broccoli)*, since they may reduce the efficacy of the prescription.

10. Unpasteurized Foods and Beverages: Bacterial contamination may occur in unpasteurized dairy products, juices, and other beverages. Choose pasteurised products instead.

11. Too much caffeine: Although some people may tolerate a modest amount of caffeine, too much of it might dehydrate you and interfere with your sleep.

12. Excessive Salt and High-Sodium Condiments: Steer clear of sprinkling excess salt on your food and exercise caution when using high-sodium condiments like ketchup, soy sauce and pickles.

FOODS TO EMBRACE IN YOUR DIET

Your food decisions may impact how well your body heals, prevent problems and support your immune system. The following foods should be a part of your diet after a liver transplant:

Foods high in protein: Protein is necessary for immune system health, muscle mass maintenance, and tissue repair. Choose lean protein sources, such as tofu and tempeh, as well as skinless chicken, fish, eggs, lentils, low-fat dairy products and fish.

High-Fiber Foods: Fibre maintains gut health, assists in digestion, and prevents constipation. Pick whole grains like whole wheat pasta, brown rice, quinoa and whole grain bread. To receive a range of minerals and antioxidants, including a variety of fruits and vegetables *(avoid those with high vitamin K content if you are on blood thinners).*

Include healthy fat sources like avocados, nuts, seeds, olive oil and fatty fish *(such as salmon, mackerel and sardines)* that are high in omega-3 fatty acids in your diet. These lipids are advantageous for reducing general inflammation and maintaining heart function.

Reduce your salt consumption to promote healthy blood pressure and avoid fluid retention by choosing low-sodium foods. Avoid packaged and processed foods since they often contain a lot of salt. Use herbs, spices, lemon juice, and other salt-free seasonings to season your food instead.

Vitamins and minerals: To acquire the vital vitamins *(such vitamins A, C, and E)* and minerals *(including potassium and magnesium)*, eat a range of colourful fruits and vegetables. These nutrients are essential for maintaining a healthy immune system and body.

Drink plenty of fluids to support digestion and help your body heal. The best option is water, but you may also consume hydrating foods like cucumbers and melons, herbal teas and fruit drinks that have been diluted.

Limit your consumption of sugar and processed meals since they may stress your liver and increase your risk of developing insulin resistance. Pick complete, unadulterated meals wherever possible and consume less sweet snacks, sweets and drinks.

Foods High in Iron: Iron is essential for the development of red blood cells and general energy levels. Include both heme *(found in lean meats and poultry)* and non-heme *(found in plant-based sources including beans, lentils, fortified cereals and spinach)* sources of iron. Iron absorption may be improved by eating foods high in vitamin C coupled with sources of iron.

Calcium and vitamin D: Calcium is essential for strong bones, while vitamin D helps the body absorb calcium. Include low-fat dairy products, fortified plant-based milk substitutes, leafy greens and exposure to sunshine for vitamin D production, depending on your particular requirements and medical recommendations.

Supplements should be used with caution: While some individuals may benefit from taking supplements, it's important to speak with your doctor first. Some supplements may interfere with certain drugs or affect how well your liver functions.

Herbal treatments and dietary supplements should be used with caution since some of them may interact with certain pharmaceuticals and impair liver function. Before incorporating any new supplements into your regimen, always check with your healthcare provider.

Gradual Changes and Monitoring: Your body may need some time to adapt to dietary changes after a liver transplant. Change your dietary habits gradually and pay attention to how your body reacts. Observe any changes in your digestion, level of energy and general wellbeing.

Maintain a Healthy Weight: A healthy weight may be attained by following a balanced diet and engaging in regular physical exercise. The liver may be overworked and negatively impacted by both quick weight reduction and severe weight gain.

Cleanliness and Food Safety: To reduce the danger of contracting foodborne infections, it's essential to adhere to stringent cleanliness and food safety procedures given that immune-suppressing drugs are often provided after transplant.

Customised Meal Planning: Develop a meal plan that is suited to your individual requirements by working with a licenced dietitian. Your meals will benefit your recovery if you can handle any dietary restrictions, allergies and sensitivities you may have.

Blood tests are frequently performed by your medical team to check your nutritional levels and liver function. This information will direct any dietary and supplement changes that are required.

Emotional Well-being and Mindful Eating: The process of healing greatly depends on psychological well-being. Your entire health and recovery may be aided by mindful eating techniques and a pleasant connection with food.

Your effective rehabilitation and enhanced quality of life will be significantly influenced by a nutritious diet and a balanced lifestyle. Open communication with your medical team, which includes your transplant surgeon, hepatologist, dietician and other experts, is crucial. You can promote the health of your new liver by adhering to their advice and eating a balanced, nutrient-rich diet.

CHAPTER 6:

DEALING WITH DIGESTIVE ISSUES

Probiotics and Gut Health Support:

Live bacteria known as probiotics have been shown to have positive effects on health when taken in sufficient quantities. Because it is thought that they assist in maintaining a healthy microbial habitat in the gut, which is crucial for general digestive and immunological function, they are often referred to as "good" or "friendly" bacteria.

A diverse community of microbes, comprising different types of bacteria, viruses, fungus and other microbes, makes up the gut microbiota. These microbes must coexist in a healthy balance for optimal digestion, food absorption, immune system control and even mental wellness.

Probiotics are present in many foods and dietary supplements. Typical probiotic sources include:

Probiotics are often found in yoghurt, especially strains of Lactobacillus and Bifidobacterium.

Foods that have been fermented, such as kimchi, sauerkraut, kefir and kombucha, also contain active probiotic bacteria.

Supplements: Each formulation of probiotic supplements has a unique strain of bacteria. It's crucial to choose supplements that have undergone thorough study and have strains that address your particular health issues.

Probiotics may have the following advantages and play a supportive role in gut health:

Digestive Health: Probiotics may assist in maintaining a balanced population of gut bacteria, which can improve digestion and relieve symptoms of IBS, diarrhoea and constipation.

Support for the immune system: The gut is home to a major percentage of the immune system. Probiotics may contribute to the control of immunological responses and the improvement of the body's defences.

Reduced Inflammation: Specific probiotic strains have been associated with decreased intestinal inflammation, which is advantageous for diseases like inflammatory bowel disease *(IBD)*.

Nutrient Absorption: By dissolving complex substances that the body would find challenging to digest on its own, certain probiotics might improve nutrient absorption.

The gut-brain axis, which is a term that has recently gained popularity, has been linked to mental health. Probiotics may help to maintain mental health and may even lessen the signs of anxiety and despair.

While probiotics have shown encouraging outcomes in a number of studies, it's crucial to remember that further study is still required to completely understand their methods of action and their impact on certain health issues. It's a good idea to speak with a healthcare provider if you're thinking about incorporating probiotics into your routine, particularly if you have any underlying medical issues.

Take into account the following factors while choosing a probiotic supplement:

Diversity of Strains: Look for items that include a range of well studied strains. Colony-Forming Units or CFUs, are a measure of how many live bacteria are present in a product. The ideal dose might change according to the demands of the person; more CFUs are not necessarily better.

Efficacy and research Select goods that have been proven effective in clinical studies and are supported by science. Handling and storing Live organisms known as probiotics are susceptible to heat and dampness.

Follow the manufacturer's recommendations for safe storage. *Keep in mind that each person's response to probiotics will be unique, and what works for one person may not necessarily work the same way for another. Overall gut health is also influenced by a healthy lifestyle and a balanced, high-fibre diet*.

RECIPES:

QUICK AND EASY RECIPES FOR BUSY DAYS

Here are a few fast, simple, and perfect for hectic days meals that are kind to the liver:

Plain Muesli:

Ingredients:

- Oats, rolled, in a cup
- 1 cup of water or low-fat milk
- Honey or bananas that have been mashed up ripley
- Cinnamon, if desired

Instructions:

In a bowl that can be microwaved, combine the oats and milk/water.

Stirring once or twice throughout the first two to three minutes on high. If you want it sweeter, add honey or mashed banana. You may also add cinnamon, if you want.

Vegetable stir-fry

Ingredients:

- Bell peppers, broccoli, carrots, zucchini, and other colourful veggies
- Lean protein *(turkey, tofu and chicken)*
- Healthy stir-fry sauce

Instructions:

Over medium-high heat, preheat a nonstick pan.

When the protein is almost through cooking, add it and put aside. Stir-fry the veggies in the skillet until they are just beginning to soften.

Return the stir-fry sauce, return the protein back to the pan and simmer for an additional few minutes.

The Quinoa salad

Ingredients:

- Prepared quinoa
- Chopped fresh veggies *(such as red onion, tomato, and cucumber).*
- Fresh herbs, chopped *(parsley, mint, basil)*
- Dressing made with lemon juice and olive oil

Instructions:

In a bowl, combine cooked quinoa with chopped veggies and herbs.

Olive oil and lemon juice should be drizzled over. Combine by tossing.

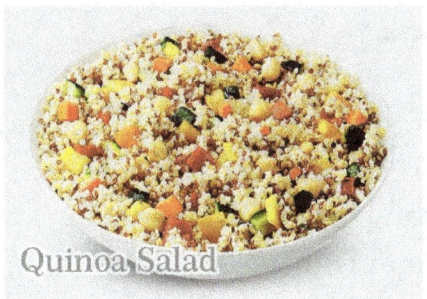

Sweet Potatoes mashed:

Ingredients:

- Sweet potatoes cooked
- Greek yoghurt with little fat
- The cinnamon spice
- A little amount of maple syrup

Instructions:

With a fork, mash cooked sweet potatoes.

Add Greek yoghurt, a dash of cinnamon, and, if preferred, a little maple syrup to the mixture.

Easy Fish Bake:

Ingredients:

- White fish fillet, such as cod or tilapia
- Citrus juice
- Fresh herbs *(parsley, dill)*
- Almond oil

- Pepper and salt

Instructions:

Set the oven's temperature to 375°F (190°C).

The fish fillet should be put on a baking sheet. Sprinkle with herbs, salt and pepper, then drizzle with olive oil and lemon juice.

Bake the fish for 15 to 20 minutes or until it flakes easily with a fork.

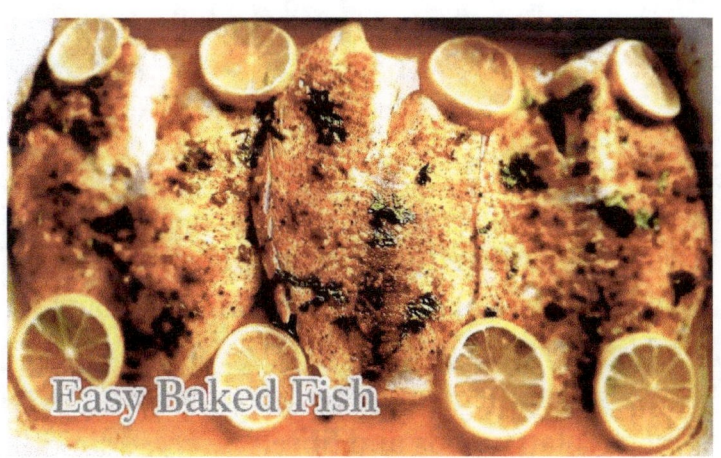

BREAKFAST AND BRUNCH RECIPES

Fresh Berries and Muesli:

- To make rolled oats creamy, add water or milk *(dairy or plant-based)*.
- Add fresh mixed berries *(blueberries, strawberries and raspberries)* on top for fibre and antioxidants.
- For additional flavour and nutrition, sprinkle chopped nuts *(such as almonds or walnuts)* or pour honey over the dish.

Greek yoghurt dessert

Greek yoghurt reduced in fat is layered with low sugar granola and sliced mango, banana, and kiwi fruits.
Add a spoonful of chia seeds on top for more omega-3 fatty acids and fibre.

Omelette with Vegetables:

- Eggs or egg whites are whisked with a little milk.
- In olive oil, cook diced veggies *(such as bell peppers, spinach, tomatoes and onions)* until they are soft.
- When the egg mixture is ready, pour it over the veggies and simmer it.
- Serve with a side of fresh fruit or whole-grain bread.

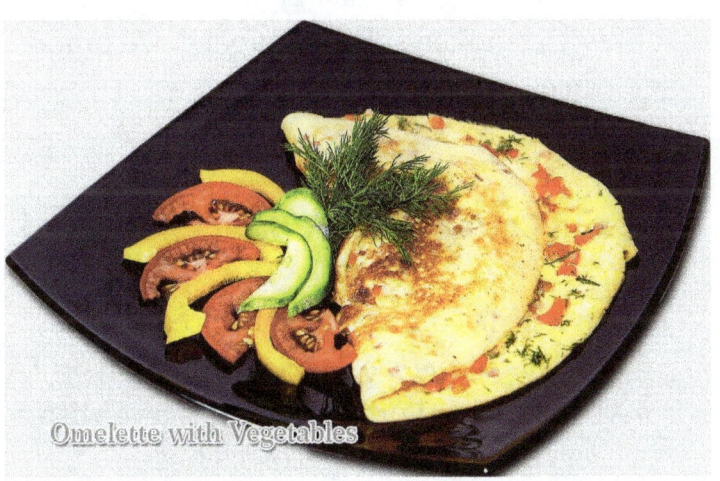

Wholesome Pancakes

Make pancakes using oat or whole wheat flour. Sliced bananas, low-fat yoghurt and pure maple syrup should be drizzled on top.

Toasted Smoked Salmon:

- Cream cheese or mashed avocado may be spread over whole grain bread.
- For a filling and tasty alternative, top with smoked salmon, capers, red onion slices and fresh dill.

Fruit and Cottage Cheese Salad:

- In a dish, combine several fresh fruits *(melon, pineapple, berries and grapes)*.
- For an added protein boost, serve with a serving of low-fat cottage cheese.

Breakfast Burrito with Veggies:

- Sauteed spinach, bell peppers and zucchini with scrambled eggs.
- The egg and vegetable combination should be placed into a whole-wheat tortilla.
- Add some salsa and a sprinkling of shredded cheese.

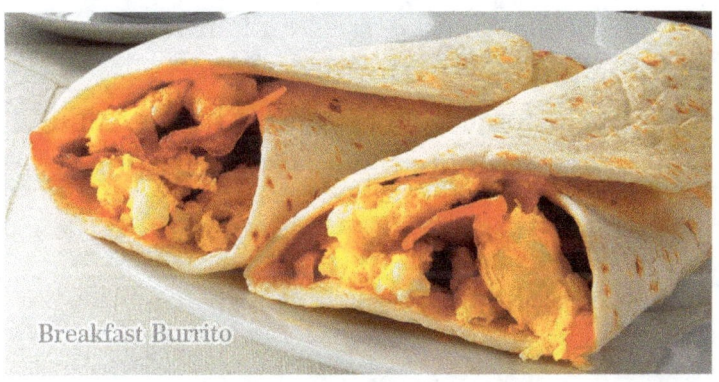

Breakfast Burrito

Blender Bowl:

- Blend frozen fruits *(mango, berries and banana)* with a little milk or a dairy-free substitute.

- Place the smoothie in a bowl and sprinkle with granola, almond slices and coconut flakes for decoration.

Breakfast bowl with Quinoa:

- Quinoa should be prepared as directed on the packaging.
- Add chopped nuts, dried fruit *(such as raisins or cranberries)* and either honey or cinnamon to the top.
- Add some finely chopped fresh fruit as well for more flavour and nutrition.

Make-Your-Own Breakfast Burrito:

- Scrambled eggs, black beans, chopped tomatoes and a sprinkling of low-fat cheese should all be placed within a whole-grain tortilla.
- Enjoy a meal that's high in protein by rolling it up.

Chia Seed Dessert:

- Combine chia seeds with a little vanilla essence and the milk of your choosing, whether it be dairy or plant-based.
- Overnight in the refrigerator will help it thicken.
- Add sliced almonds, fresh berries and a sprinkle of pure maple syrup to the top in the morning.

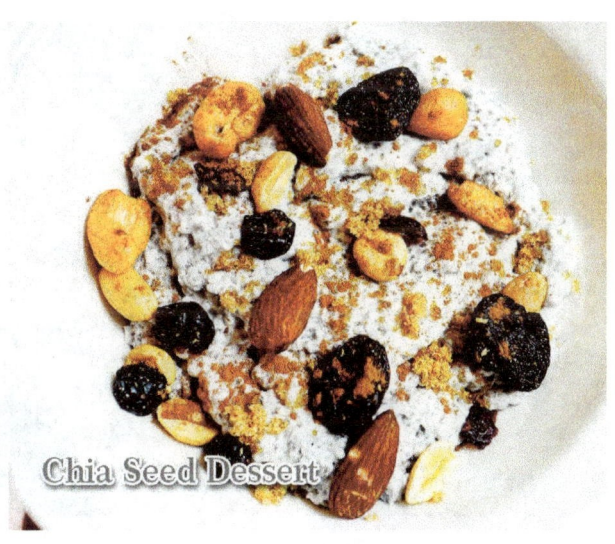

Frittata with Spinach and Mushrooms:

- With a little milk, whisk eggs or egg whites.
- In hot olive oil, cook mushrooms and spinach until they are soft.
- When the egg mixture is ready, pour it over the vegetables.
- Serving with a side salad after being cut into wedges.

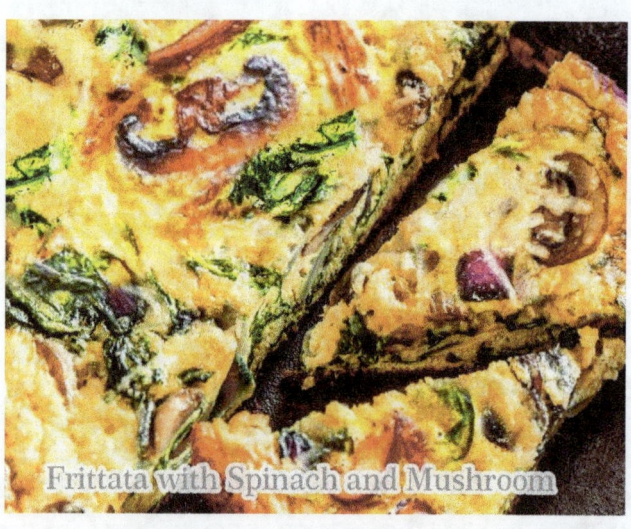
Frittata with Spinach and Mushroom

Morning Smoothie:

- Leafy greens *(such as spinach or kale)*, a selection of fruits, a scoop of protein powder, and a liquid base *(milk, yoghurt, or a dairy-free substitute)* should all be blended together.
- A tablespoon of nut butter may be added for more protein and good fats.

Poached Egg on Avocado Toast:

- Put ripe avocado over whole grain bread and mash it.
- Add a poached egg, some salt, pepper and chopped parsley or chives as garnishes.

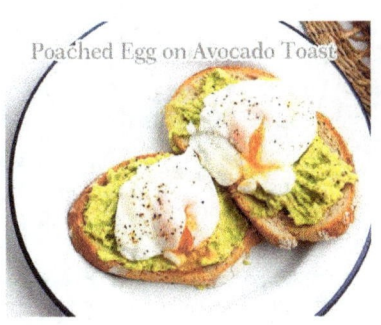

Banana and Nut Butter on Rice Cakes:

- Rice cakes should be covered with natural nut butter, such as almond or peanut butter.
- Slices of banana with honey drizzled on top.

Authentic Muesli:

- Rollin oats, chopped nuts, seeds *(such as sunflower or pumpkin seeds)*, dried fruit and a little cinnamon should all be combined.
- Serve with milk or yoghurt of your choice.

LUNCH AND DINNER RECIPES

Lunch Meals:

Salad with Grilled Chicken:

Over mixed greens with tomatoes, cucumbers, and a mild vinaigrette, grilled chicken breast is served.

Cooking Guidelines: Marinate chicken in a mixture of lemon juice, herbs, garlic and olive oil. Cook completely on the grill.

Stir-fry with Quinoa and Vegetables:

Bell peppers, broccoli, and other vibrant veggies are stir-fried with quinoa.

Cooking Guidelines: Quinoa should be prepared as directed on the packaging. Using a little oil, stir-fry some chopped vegetables while seasoning with low-sodium soy sauce.

Bean Soup:

A filling lentil soup cooked with veggies and a broth low in salt.

Instructions for cooking: Sauté celery, onions, and carrots. Add broth and cleaned lentils. Till lentils are cooked, simmer.

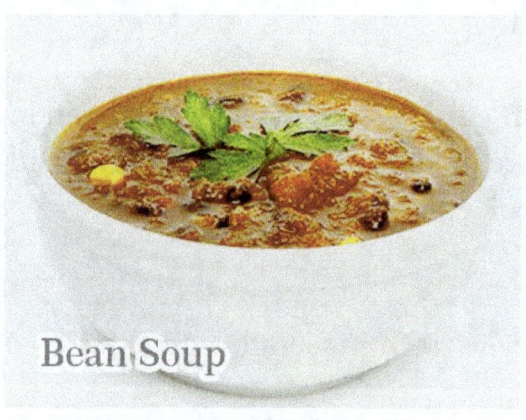

Salmon Baked with Roasted Veggies:
Roasted sweet potatoes, Brussels sprouts and asparagus are paired with baked salmon fillet.

Cooking Instructions: Salmon should be baked after being herb-seasoned.
Vegetables should be seasoned, then roasted in olive oil until soft.

Turkey Sandwich:
Slices of lean turkey, lettuce, tomatoes and hummus are all wrapped in whole wheat.

Cooking instructions: Put the stuff you want in the wrap.

Salad with Avocado and Turkey:

Lean turkey slices, avocado, mixed greens, cherry tomatoes and a dressing made with lemon and tahini.

Cooking Guidelines: With the aforementioned components, assemble the salad and top with the dressing.

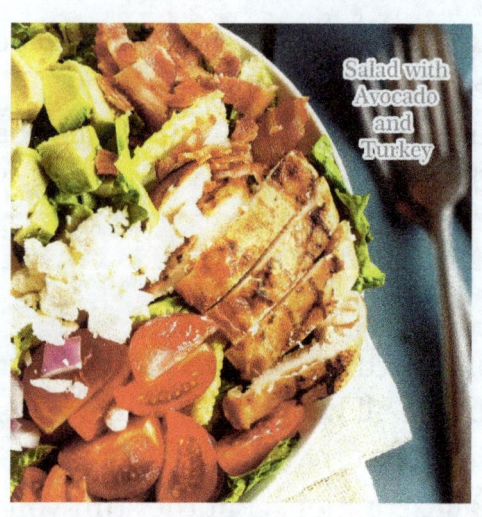

Salad with Avocado and Turkey

Chickpea and Veggie Curry:

Brown rice is served with a delicious curry cooked with a variety of veggies and chickpeas.

Cooking Guidelines: Sauté curry spices, onions, and garlic. Add coconut milk, chickpeas, and chopped vegetables. Simmer the veggies until they are ready.

Wrap with Grilled Veggies:

Grilled veggies with a mild yoghurt-based sauce *(such as bell peppers, zucchini, and eggplant)* wrapped in a whole wheat tortilla.

Cooking Guidelines: After grilling the veggies, put the sauce on the wrap.

Cod in the oven with Quinoa Pilaf:

Quinoa pilaf with plenty of vegetables and baked fish fillet with a lemon-dill sauce.

Cooking Guidelines: Cod is baked with quinoa prepared as directed on the box and veggies that have been sautéed.

Grilled Chicken served with a Spinach and Berry Salad:

Grilled chicken, baby spinach, mixed berries, sliced almonds and balsamic vinaigrette.

Cooking Guidelines: Assemble the salad using the aforementioned ingredients and grill the chicken.

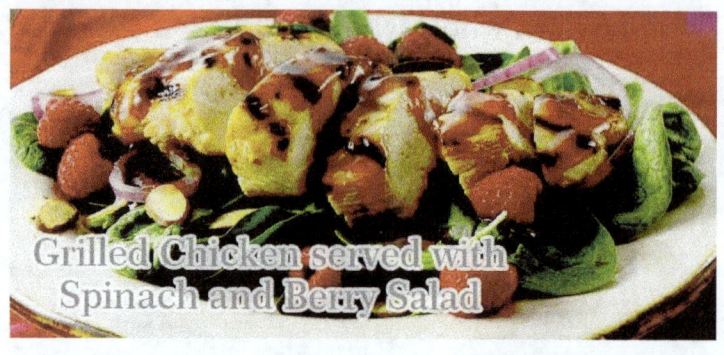
Grilled Chicken served with Spinach and Berry Salad

Quinoa Caprese Salad

Cherry tomatoes, fresh mozzarella, basil leaves, and a splash of balsamic glaze are combined with quinoa.

Cooking Guidelines: Halved cherry tomatoes, mozzarella balls, and torn basil leaves are added to cooked quinoa. Apply a balsamic glaze.

White Fish Grilled with Steaming Broccoli:

Served with steamed broccoli, fresh lemon juice and broiled white fish with herbs and lemon.

Cooking Guidelines: Fish fillet should be seasoned before broiling. Lemon juice is used to season the steamed broccoli.

Stir-fry with Vegetables and Tofu:

Brown rice is served with tofu that has been stir-fried with a variety of bell peppers, snow peas, carrots and a ginger-soy sauce.

Cooking instructions: Tofu and vegetables to be stir-fried before sauce is added and brown rice is prepared.

Chicken Salad with Greek Yoghurt:

Greek yoghurt, diced celery, grapes and chopped walnuts are combined with shredded chicken and served in lettuce cups.

Cooking Instructions: Prepare chicken by cooking and shredding it. Combine chicken with yoghurt, sliced celery, quartered grapes and chopped walnuts. Use lettuce cups to serve.

Frittata with Vegetables:

A meal of baked eggs with sautéed veggies, such spinach, bell peppers and onions, with feta cheese on top.

Cooking directions: Saute vegetables, stir in beaten eggs, bake until set, then top with feta.

Salad of Chicken with Walnuts:

Over a bed of mixed greens with dried cranberries and a mild vinaigrette, chicken breast is baked with crumbled walnuts on top.

Cooking Guidelines: Crush walnuts to coat the chicken, then bake it until done. Combine greens, cranberries and vinaigrette to make a salad.

Soup Minestrone:

A filling minestrone soup made with whole wheat pasta, beans and veggies.

Cooking Guidelines: Add pasta, beans, broth, and sautéed vegetables. Simmer the spaghetti until it is done.

White Bean and Tuna Salad:

White beans, cherry tomatoes, red onion, parsley and a lemon-olive oil vinaigrette are combined with tuna.

Cooking Guidelines: Combine the washed beans, halved tomatoes, chopped onion and parsley with the drained tuna. Dress with a drizzle.

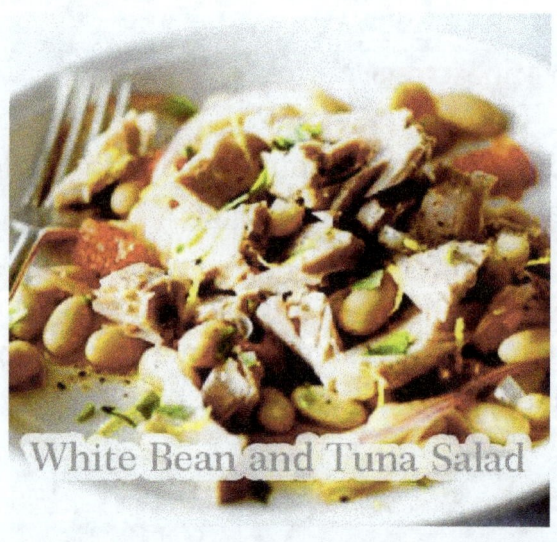
White Bean and Tuna Salad

Quesadilla with Grilled Vegetables and Goat Cheese:

Goat cheese melted between whole wheat tortillas with grilled veggies.

Cooking Guidelines: After assembling the quesadilla, grill the veggies until the cheese is melted.

Sweet & Sour Chicken baked:

Steamed jasmine rice is served with baked chicken pieces that have been covered in a handmade sweet and sour sauce.

Cooking directions call for baking the chicken pieces, making the sauce and serving it with cooked rice.

Chickpea Wrap from the Mediterranean:

Hummus, chickpeas, tomatoes, red onion, sliced cucumbers and feta cheese are all combined in a whole wheat wrap.

Cooking Guidelines: With the aforementioned components, assemble the wrap.

Quinoa Bowl with Grilled Vegetables and Feta:

Grilled veggies, feta crumbles and a lemon-oregano dressing are added to quinoa.

Cooking Guidelines: Prepare the quinoa and grill the veggies. Put the feta and dressing in the bowl.

Salmon Teriyaki with Steamed Bok Choy:

Salmon fillet with a teriyaki glaze served with brown rice and steaming bok cabbage.

Cooking Guidelines: Bake fish with a teriyaki glaze. Cook brown rice while steaming bok choy.

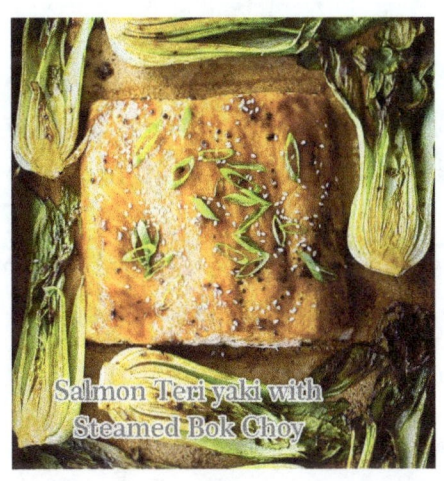
Salmon Teriyaki with Steamed Bok Choy

Salad with Mixed Beans:

A vibrant salad with a combination of maize, bell peppers, red onion, black beans, kidney beans and black beans.

Cooking Guidelines: Combine the corn, onion, peppers and beans that have been washed and drained. Mix in the dressing.

Primavera Pasta with Pesto:

Seasonal veggies are sautéed and mixed with whole wheat spaghetti in a light pesto sauce.

Prepare spaghetti, sauté vegetables and combine with pesto sauce.

Dinner Meals:

Quinoa and Grilled Vegetable Bowl:

Over quinoa, grilled zucchini, eggplant and red onion are presented.

Cooking Guidelines: Separately cooking the quinoa and grilling the veggies. Combine and add olive oil as a drizzle.

Tofu in a Stir-fry with Brown Rice:

Over brown rice, tofu is stir-fried with bell peppers, broccoli and snap peas.

Cooking Guidelines: Put tofu in a thin sauce to marinate. Serve tofu and vegetables over cooked brown rice after stir-frying.

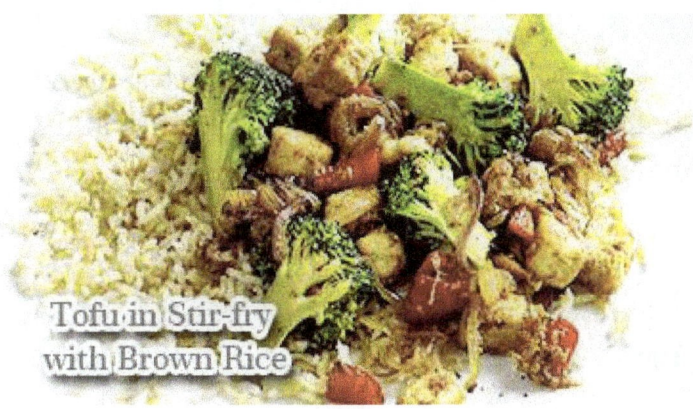

Tofu in Stir-fry with Brown Rice

Steamed Green Beans with Baked Chicken:

Served with steaming green beans is a chicken thigh that has been baked with garlic and rosemary.

Cooking Guidelines: Bake chicken after seasoning. To make green beans tender, steam them.

Bean and Vegetable Stew:

A filling stew made with kidney beans, assorted veggies, and a tomato-based broth.

Cooking Guidelines: Vegetables are sautéed before being combined with the broth and beans.

Pork Chops on the Grill with Mashed Cauliflower:

Herb-seasoned, grilled pork chops with mashed cauliflower as a side dish.

Cooking Guidelines: Cook mashed cauliflower *(steam cauliflower, mash and season)* while grilling pork chops.

Stir-fried Prawns with Rice Noodles:

Rice noodles are stir-fried in a ginger-soy sauce with shrimp, colourful bell peppers, snap peas and other vegetables.

Cooking Guidelines: Shrimp and vegetables are stir-fried before rice noodles and sauce are added.

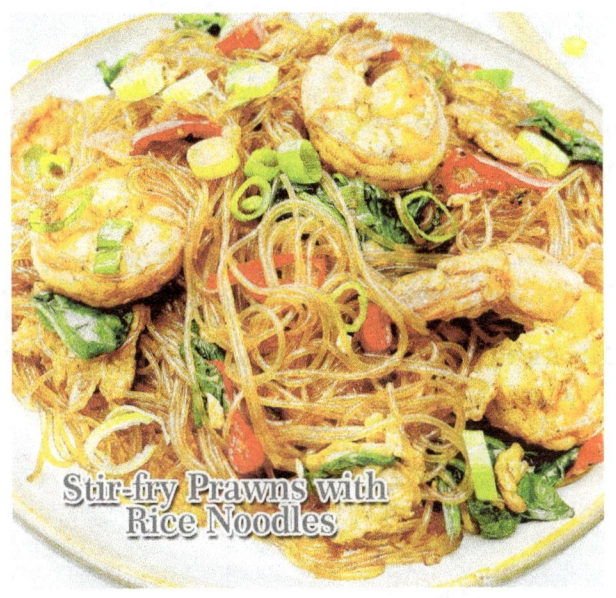

Stir-fry Prawns with Rice Noodles

Sweet Potato mash with Roasted Turkey:

Roasted turkey breast with steaming green beans and creamy sweet potato mash.

Cooking Guidelines: Prepare sweet potatoes *(boil, mash and season)* and roast the turkey.

Chickpea Salad from the Mediterranean:

Chickpeas, cucumbers, red onions, Kalamata olives, feta cheese and a lemon-oregano vinaigrette makeup this light salad.

Cooking Guidelines: With the aforementioned components, assemble the salad and top with the dressing.

Eggplant Parmesan in a bake:

With whole wheat spaghetti, cooked breaded eggplant slices are topped with layers of marinara sauce and mozzarella cheese.

Cooking Guidelines: Layers of eggplant are assembled, breaded and baked until the cheese is melted.

Steak on the Grill with Roasted Root Vegetables:

roasted potatoes, carrots, and parsnips well with grilled steak that has been marinated in rosemary and garlic.

Cooking Guidelines: Grill or marinate the meat, roast the root vegetables and season the marinated beef.

Grilled Halibut with Lemon and Herbs and Couscous:

Lemon-infused couscous and steamed asparagus are served with grilled halibut that has been seasoned with lemon and herbs.

Cooking Guidelines: Halibut on the grill with lemon and herbs, precooked couscous and steamed asparagus.

Quinoa and Ratatouille:

With cooked quinoa, ratatouille is produced with eggplant, zucchini, bell peppers, tomatoes and herbs.

Cooking Guidelines: Vegetables are sautéed before tomatoes and herbs are added and the flavours are blended. Over cooked quinoa, serve.

Baked Bell Peppers With Stuffing:

Lean ground turkey, brown rice, tomatoes and seasonings filled within bell peppers.

Cooking Guidelines: Prepare the filling, stuff the peppers, and bake them until they are soft.

Stir-Fry with Lentils and Vegetables:

Over whole grain noodles, cooked lentils are stir-fried with a variety of veggies and a sesame-soy sauce.

Cooking Guidelines: Serve lentils over cooked noodles after stirring in sauce and some stir-fried vegetables.

Hummus & Grilled Veggie Wrap:

Hummus with grilled veggies *(such as zucchini, bell peppers and onions)* on a whole wheat tortilla.

Cooking Guidelines: Using grilled veggies and hummus, create the wrap.

Baked cod with Lemon and Dill and Roasted Brussels Sprouts:

Roasted Brussels sprouts are served with a baked fish fillet seasoned with lemon and dill.

Cooking Guidelines: Baked cod is seasoned with lemon and dill. Roast Brussels sprouts after tossing in olive oil.

Spinach with mushrooms Chicken breast stuffed:

Quinoa is served with chicken breast that has been filled with spinach, mushrooms and low-fat mozzarella.

Cooking Guidelines: Stuff chicken with mushrooms and spinach, then bake. Make the quinoa.

Tofu and Broccoli stir-fry with an Asian flair:

Brown rice is paired with tofu and broccoli that have been stir-fried in a delicious sesame-ginger sauce.

Cooking Guidelines: Cooked brown rice should be served with the tofu, broccoli and sauce.

Lentil and Vegetable Curry:

Warming curry with naan bread cooked with lentils, mixed veggies and flavorful spices.

Cooking Guidelines: Sauté the spices, onions, and garlic. Add the lentils, broth, and veggies. Till lentils are cooked, simmer. Toss in some naan.

Ricotta and Spinach Portobello Mushroom stuffed:

Stuffed portobello mushrooms with a blend of ricotta cheese, spinach and seasonings.

Cooking Guidelines: To fill mushrooms, combine ricotta, herbs and sautéed spinach. Bake.

Zucchini Boats Stuffed:

Slices of zucchini packed with a blend of brown rice, chopped tomatoes, seasonings and ground turkey.

Cooking Guidelines: Prepare the filling, hollow out the zucchini halves and bake until the zucchini is soft.

Tofu in a Thai Coconut Curry:

Over jasmine rice, a flavorful curry made with coconut, tofu, bell peppers, carrots and snow peas.

Cooking Guidelines: Add coconut milk and Thai curry paste after sautéing the vegetables and tofu. Over cooked jasmine rice, please.

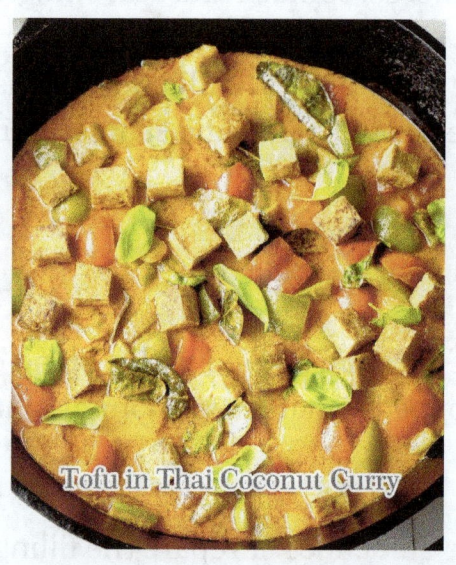

Baked Portobello Stuffed Mushrooms:

Quinoa, sautéed spinach, sun-dried tomatoes, and Parmesan cheese stuffed with portobello mushrooms.

Cooking Guidelines: Cooked quinoa, sun-dried tomatoes, and cheese are combined with sautéed spinach. Baked mushrooms with a filling.

Chicken Thighs with Herb Roast and Mashed Potatoes with Garlic:

Served with creamy garlic mashed potatoes, steaming green beans and roasted chicken thighs with fresh herbs.

Cooking Guidelines: Roast chicken after seasoning with herbs. You should boil, mash, and season potatoes. Green beans are steamed.

Quesadilla with Corn and Black Beans:

Black beans, corn, chopped tomatoes and shredded cheddar cheese are combined to fill a quesadilla.

Cooking Guidelines: Put the ingredients for the quesadilla together and heat it until the cheese is melted.

You may modify the ingredients and portion amounts of these meals to suit your own requirements and tastes. They serve as sources of inspiration. Prioritise eating a balanced diet at all times and seek personalised guidance from your doctor or a nutritionist.

SNACKS, SMOOTHIES AND DESSERTS

Snacks Meals:

Veggie Sticks and Hummus:

- On a platter, spread hummus.
- Bell peppers, cucumbers and carrots should be cut into sticks.
- Sticks are dipped into hummus.

Greek Yoghurt Dessert:

- In a glass, combine Greek yoghurt, mixed berries and a sprinkle of honey.
- Add granola on top for crunch.

Slices of Apple with Nut Butter:

- Remove the core before cutting apples.
- On each slice, spread almond or peanut butter.

Acai and Rice Cakes:

- Rice cakes should be covered with mashed avocado.
- Add a dash of salt and some red pepper flakes.

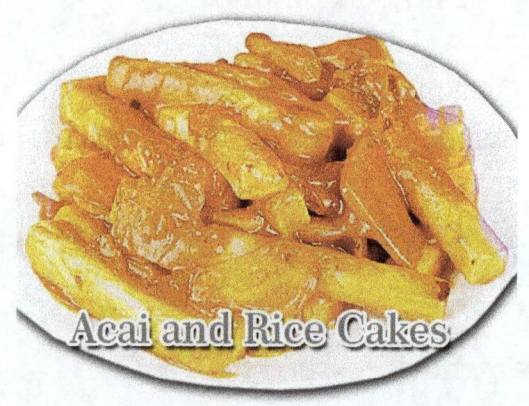

Trail Blend:

- Combine some dried fruits, unsalted almonds and dark chocolate chips.
- Place portions in little snack packs.

Guacamole and Rice Crackers:

- For a great pairing, serve rice crackers without gluten with guacamole.

Cream Cheese and Cucumber Bites:

- Sliced cucumbers are topped with a little cream cheese dollop and fresh dill.

Quinoa Salad cups:

- Prepared quinoa, chopped veggies and a little vinaigrette should be placed in lettuce cups.

Hummus and Pita with Edamame:

- Eat triangles of whole wheat pita with edamame hummus.

Rolled-up Rice paper:

- Put mint leaves, prawns, avocado, cucumber and rice paper within.
- Serve with a thin dipping sauce.

Fruits Dipped in Yoghurt:

- For a cold, creamy treat, dip fresh berries in Greek yoghurt and freeze.

Toasted Sweet Potatoes:

- Sweet potato slices are toasted, then nut butter or avocado are spread on top.

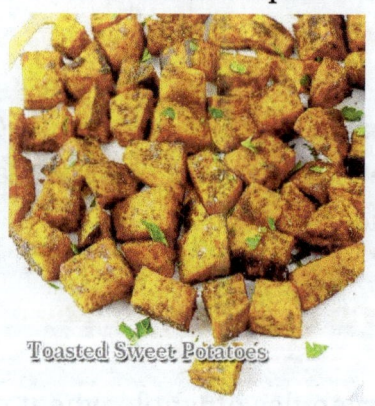
Toasted Sweet Potatoes

Pear slices with Cottage Cheese:

- Sliced ripe pears and a dollop of cottage cheese go well together.

Veggie Rice Paper Wraps:

- Julienned vegetables on rice paper with a thin hoisin dipping sauce.

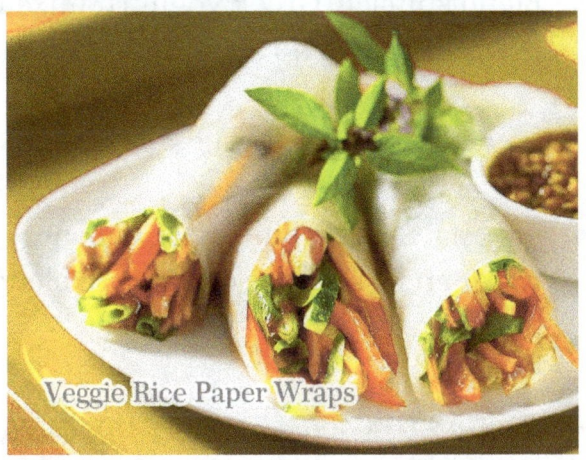

Zucchini Chips Baked in the Oven:

- Zucchini should be thinly sliced, spiced with herbs and baked until crispy.

Smoothie Meals:

Strawberry Smoothie:

- Blend spinach, Greek yoghurt, mixed berries and a little bit of almond milk.

Smoothie with Tropical Paradise:

- Banana, mango, pineapple, coconut water and a squeeze of lime are blended together.

A Green Protein Shake:

- Protein powder, spinach, banana, almond milk and a little amount of almond butter are blended together.

Blueberry and Almond Smoothie with Cream:

- Greek yoghurt, blueberries, almond milk and a few almonds should all be combined.

Banana and Peanut Butter Smoothie:

- Blend milk, banana, Greek yoghurt, peanut butter and oats.

Watermelon Cooler with Mint:

- For a cool dessert, combine watermelon, fresh mint leaves, lime juice and ice.

Smoothie with Creamy Spinach and Bananas:

- Almond milk, spinach, frozen banana and a little bit of vanilla essence are blended together.

Protein Smoothie with Chocolate and Banana:

- Blend banana, almond milk, Greek yoghurt and chocolate protein powder.

Green Smoothie with Coconut and Pineapples:

- Combining coconut milk, spinach, pineapple and a scoop of plant-based protein powder.

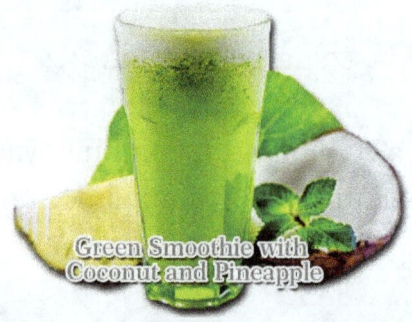

Fruity Beet Smoothie:

- Greek yoghurt, cooked beetroot, mixed berries and a little orange juice should all be combined.

Smoothie with Peach Oats:

- Blend peaches, oats, Greek yoghurt with vanilla flavour and almond milk.

Smoothie with Pumpkin Spice:

- Blend banana, coconut milk, cinnamon, nutmeg and pumpkin puree.

Smoothie with Peanut Butter Cups:

- Banana, peanut butter, almond milk and chocolate protein powder should all be blended.

Kiwi, Lime and Green Smoothie:

- Blend spinach, Greek yoghurt, kiwi, lime juice and water.

Protein Smoothie with Mango and Avocado:

- For a creamy delight, combine mango, avocado, protein powder and coconut water.

Dessert Meals:

Chia Seed Dessert:

- Almond milk, chia seeds and a little honey should be combined.
- Up until it thickens, let it rest in the refrigerator.
- Before serving, garnish with fresh fruit.

Apples Baked:

- Apples are cored, then oats, cinnamon and chopped almonds are added.
- Bake for tenderness.

Bark of Frozen Yoghurt:

- On a baking sheet, spread the Greek yoghurt.
- Strawberries, kiwis and granola sprinkles may be added as garnish.
- After freezing, splinter.

Banana-Oatmeal Cookies:

- Ripe bananas are mashed and combined with oats and a dash of cinnamon.
- Bake until golden after forming into cookies.

Dipped in Dark Chocolate Strawberries:

- Melt the bitter chocolate.
- Put strawberries on parchment paper to cool after being covered in molten chocolate.

Bites of Frozen Banana:

- Bananas should be sliced, then dipped in melted dark chocolate.
- Frozen chocolate will become more solid.

Mango Slush:

- Coconut water and frozen mango chunks should be blended until smooth.

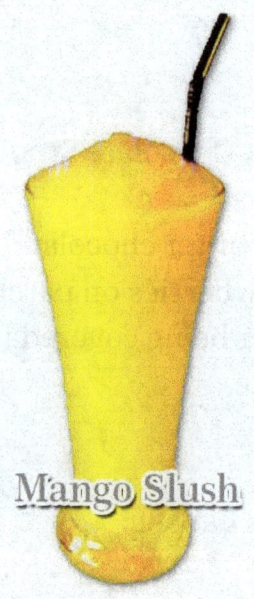
Mango Slush

Yoghurt and Pomegranate Parfait:

In a glass, combine pomegranate seeds, Greek yoghurt and a little honey.

Almonds with Cocoa Powder:

- For a chocolate crunch, toss almonds in unsweetened cocoa powder.

Nice Cream Cherry Almond:

- Almond butter, almond milk and a few frozen cherries should be blended until smooth.

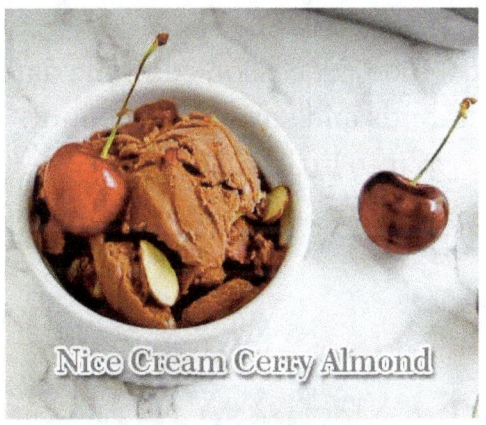

Chia-Raspberry Jam:

- Combine raspberries, chia seeds and a little honey.

- Allow it to stand until it becomes jam-like in consistency.

Banana slices with Cocoa Powder:

- Bananas are cut into slices and dusted with unsweetened chocolate powder.

Date and Almond Balls:

- In a food processor, combine dates, almonds and shredded coconut.
- Form into little balls.

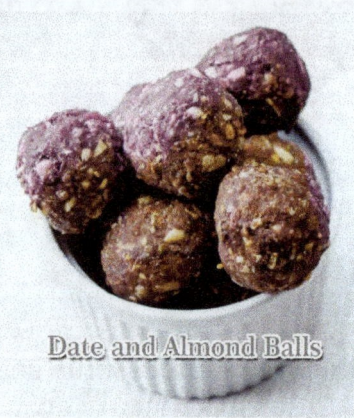
Date and Almond Balls

Yoghurt Dip with Fruit Kabobs:

- Greek yoghurt dip should be served with the skewered mixture of fruit.

Iced Yoghurt Lemon Berry Bites:

- Combine Greek yoghurt, mixed berries and lemon zest.
- Freeze after spooning into tiny muffin tins.

Bonus Recipes:

Rice Cakes with Nut Butter:
- Rice cakes should be covered in your favourite nut butter.
- For added texture, add crushed nuts to the mixture.

Fruit with Cottage Cheese:
- Sliced peaches, pineapple or berries go well with cottage cheese.

Chicken Thighs:
- Stir together the olive oil, spices and cooked chickpeas.
- Till crispy, roast.

Granola and Yoghurt Parfait:
- Your preferred yoghurt, granola and fresh fruit are layered together.

Medley of Mixed Nuts:
- For a filling snack, combine unsalted nuts like cashews, walnuts and almonds.

Seaweed Snacks:
- Graze on crisp seaweed sheets for a savoury, low-calorie snack.

Rice Cake Pizzas:
- Add tomato sauce, shredded mozzarella and your preferred vegetables to the top of the rice cakes.
- Until the cheese melts, broil.

Caprese Cherry Tomato Skewers:
- On toothpicks, attach cherry tomatoes, fresh mozzarella and basil leaves.
- Add a balsamic reduction drizzle.

Roasted Sweet Potatoes with Cinnamon:
- Sweet potato cubes should be mixed with a little cinnamon and olive oil.
- Roast until meat is tender.

Energy Bites with Fruit and Nuts:
- Combine honey, almonds and dried fruit.
- For an instant energy boost, shape into bite-sized balls.

Rice Pudding with Nuts:
- Rice should be prepared with almond milk, cinnamon and a lot of chopped almonds.

Fruit Medley With Roasts:
- With a drizzle of honey and a dusting of cinnamon, roast a variety of fruit slices.

Veggie Chips produced at home:
- Sweet potatoes, beets, or kale may be sliced thinly, drizzled with olive oil and baked until crispy.

Recall to keep up a nutritious diet that complies with your individual dietary requirements and any recommendations made by your healthcare staff.

Enjoy Your Meals
& Have a Safe Recovery

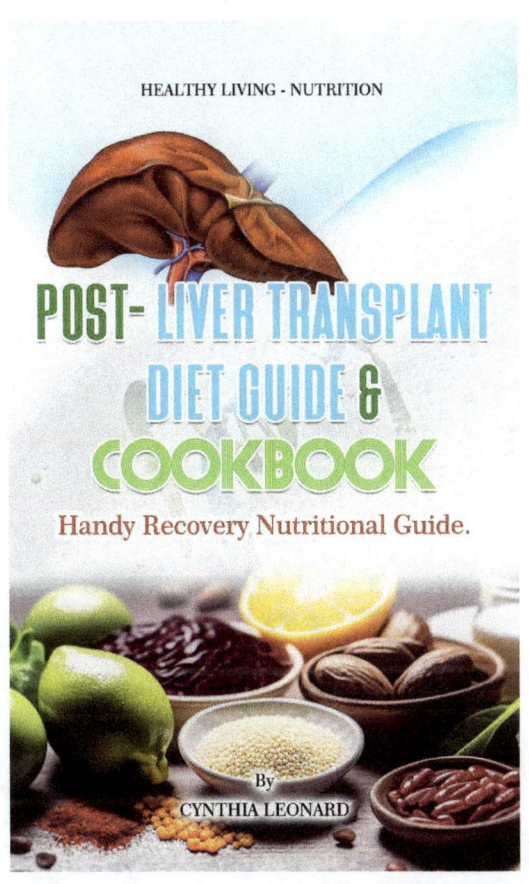

145

www.ingramcontent.com/pod-product-compliance
Lightning Source LLC
LaVergne TN
LVHW051732280225
804810LV00005B/437